Introduction

Do yoga like Abby!

I like to pose in different ways so I learn to pose the yoga way.

Follow along and see if you can do them like me.

Try the Seated Forward Fold. You can do it!

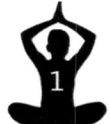

Seated Forward Fold Pose

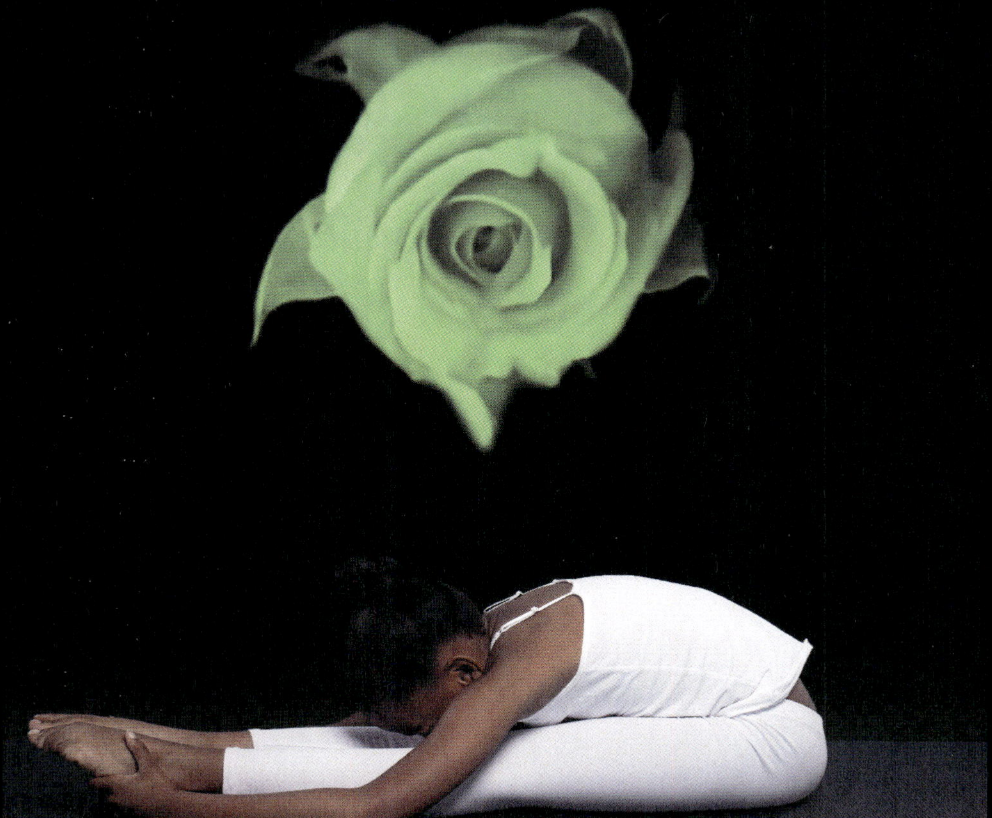

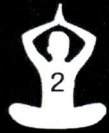

Now try the Upward Facing Dog.

I'm so proud of your yoga poses.

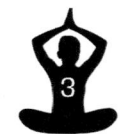

Upward Facing Dog Pose

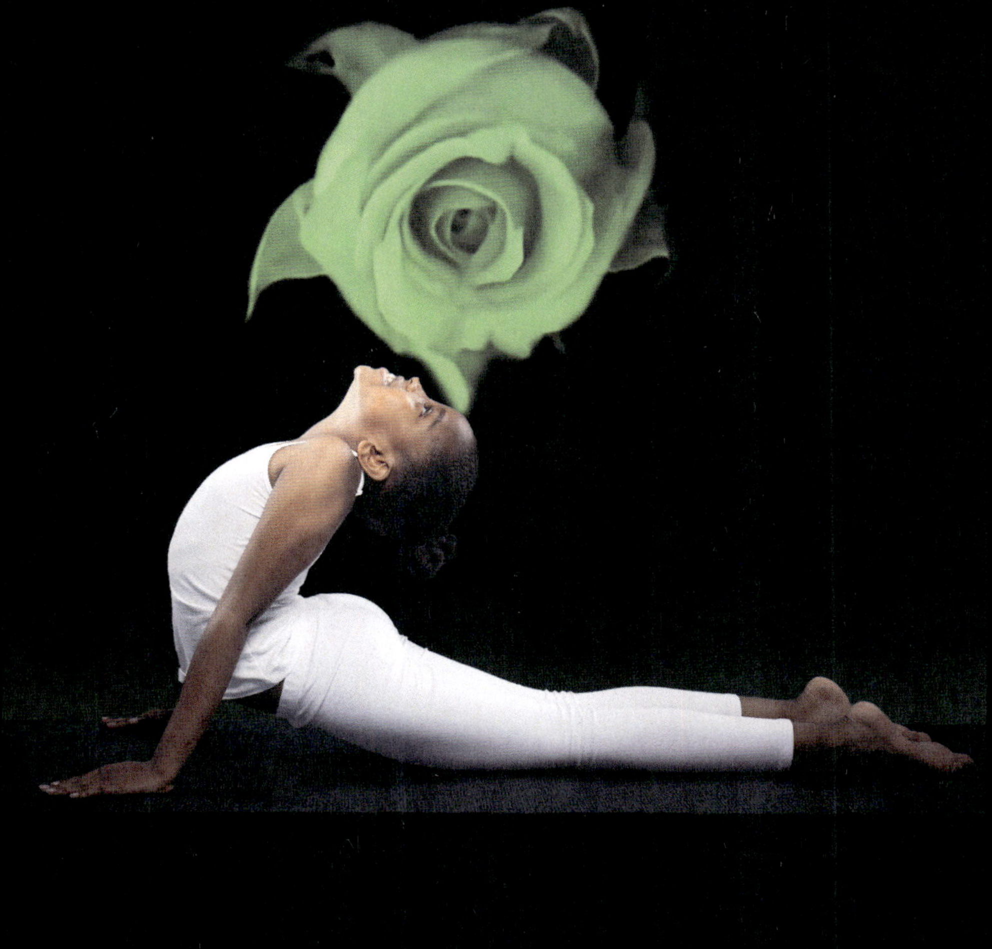

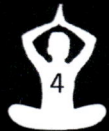

Try this next pose.

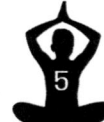

Bridge Pose

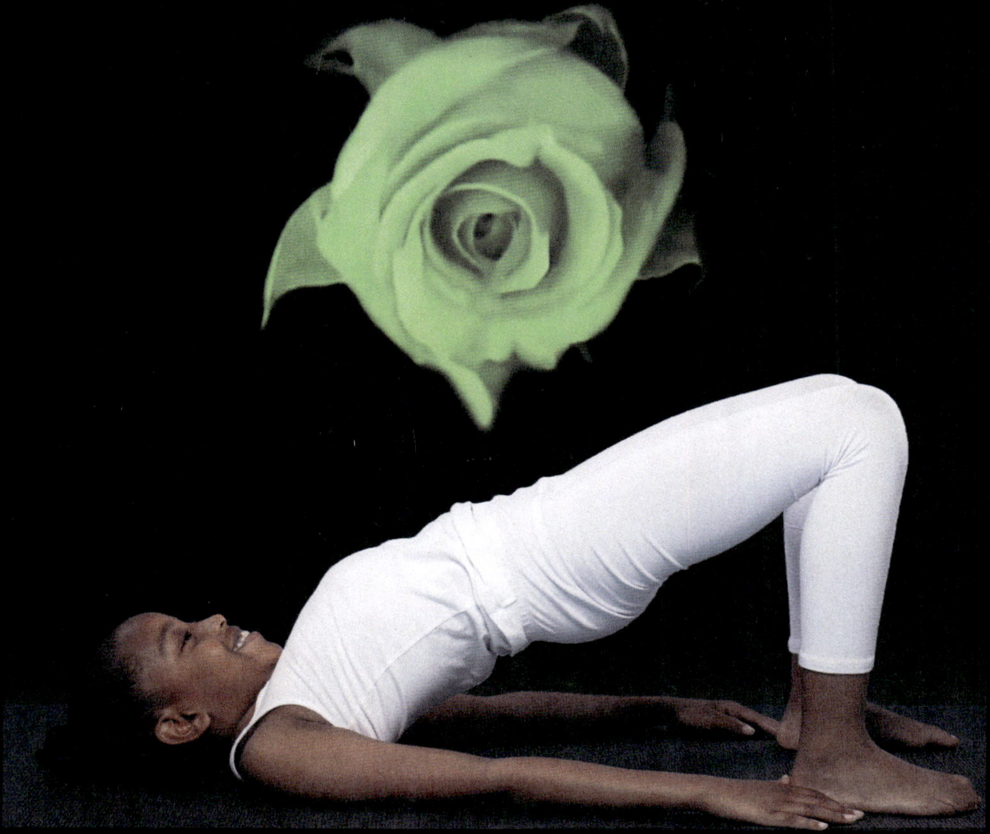

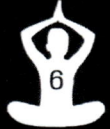

Your Yogi Squat looks perfect.

Great Job!

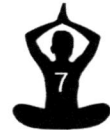

Yogi Squat Pose

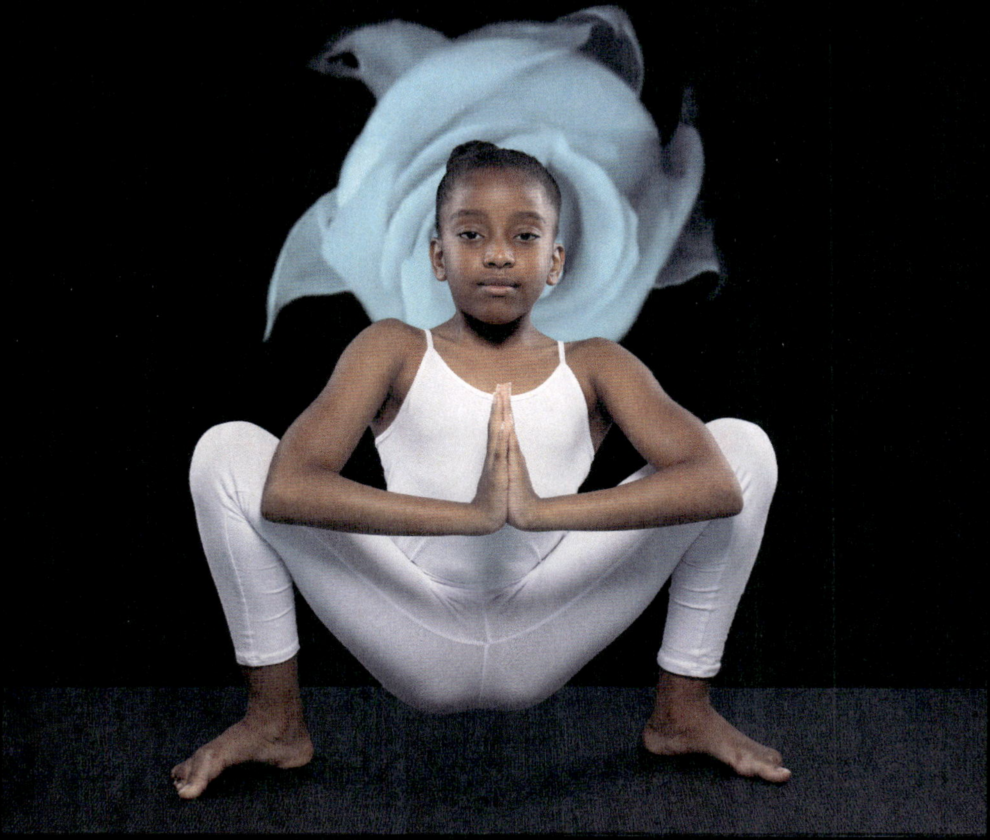

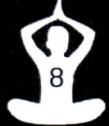

You are looking like a pro doing the Half Lord of the Fishes Pose.

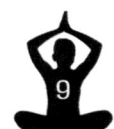

Half Lord of the Fishes Pose

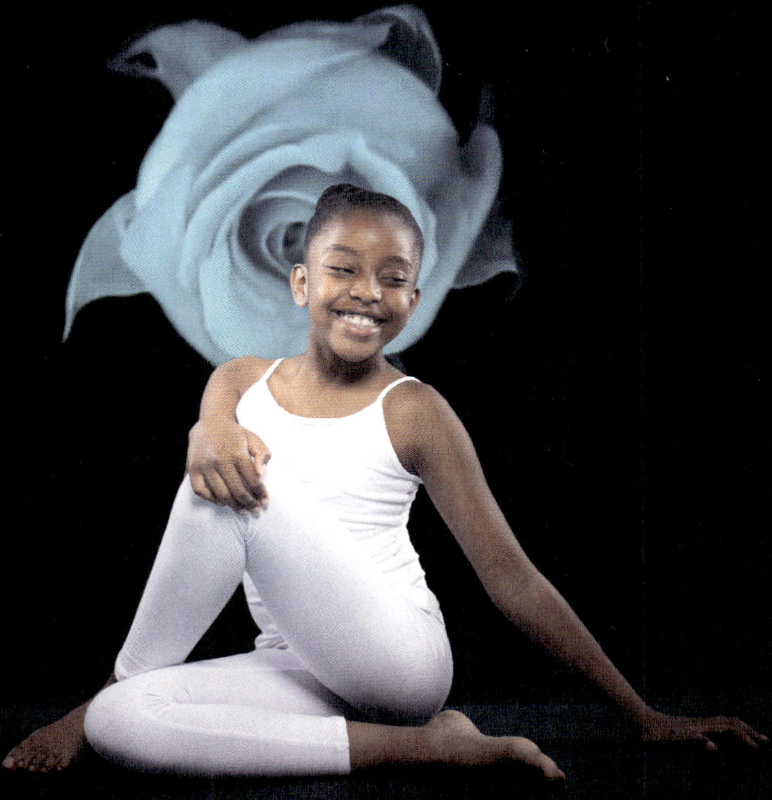

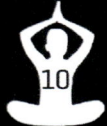

Try the One-Legged King Pigeon Pose.

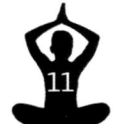

One-Legged King Pigeon Pose

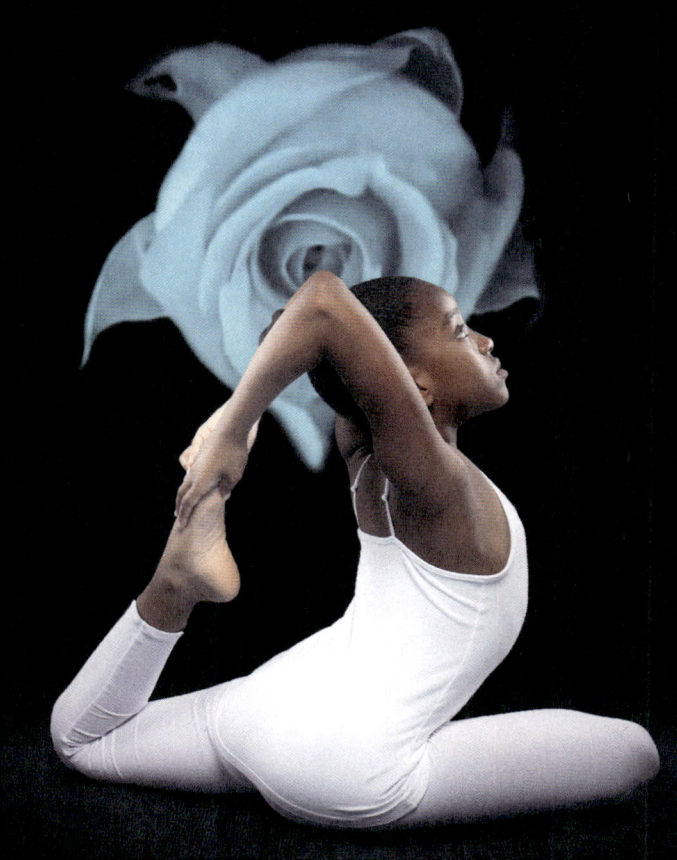

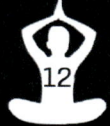

Next, try the King Cobra Pose.

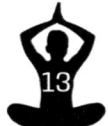

King Cobra Pose

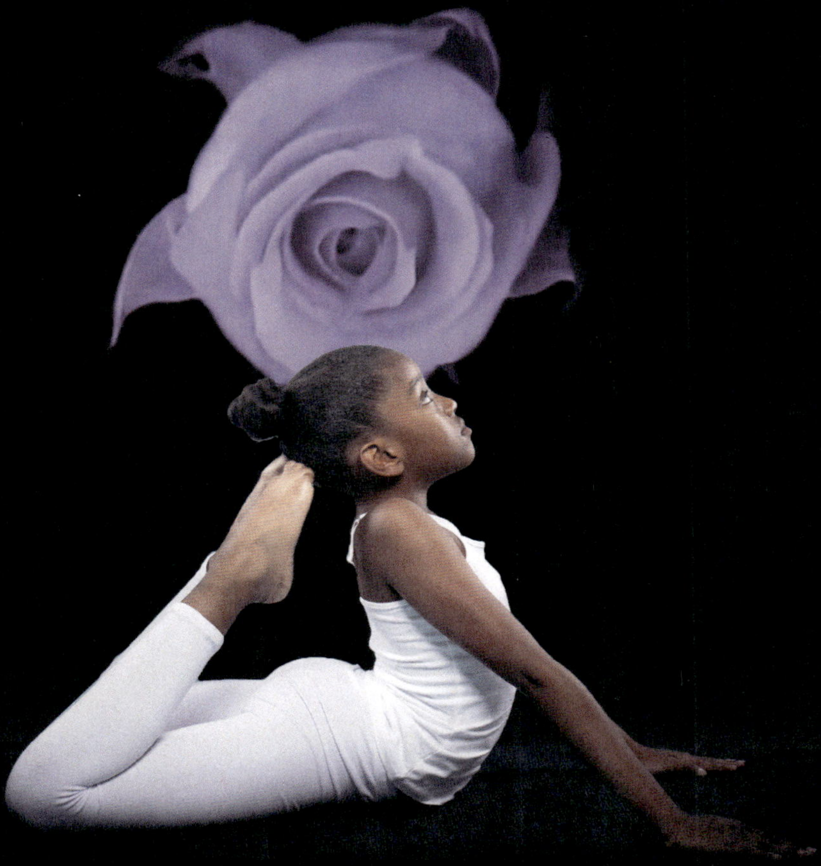

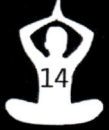

Try the King Pigeon (Kapotasana) Pose.

You're doing awesome!

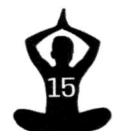

King Pigeon (Kapotasana) Pose

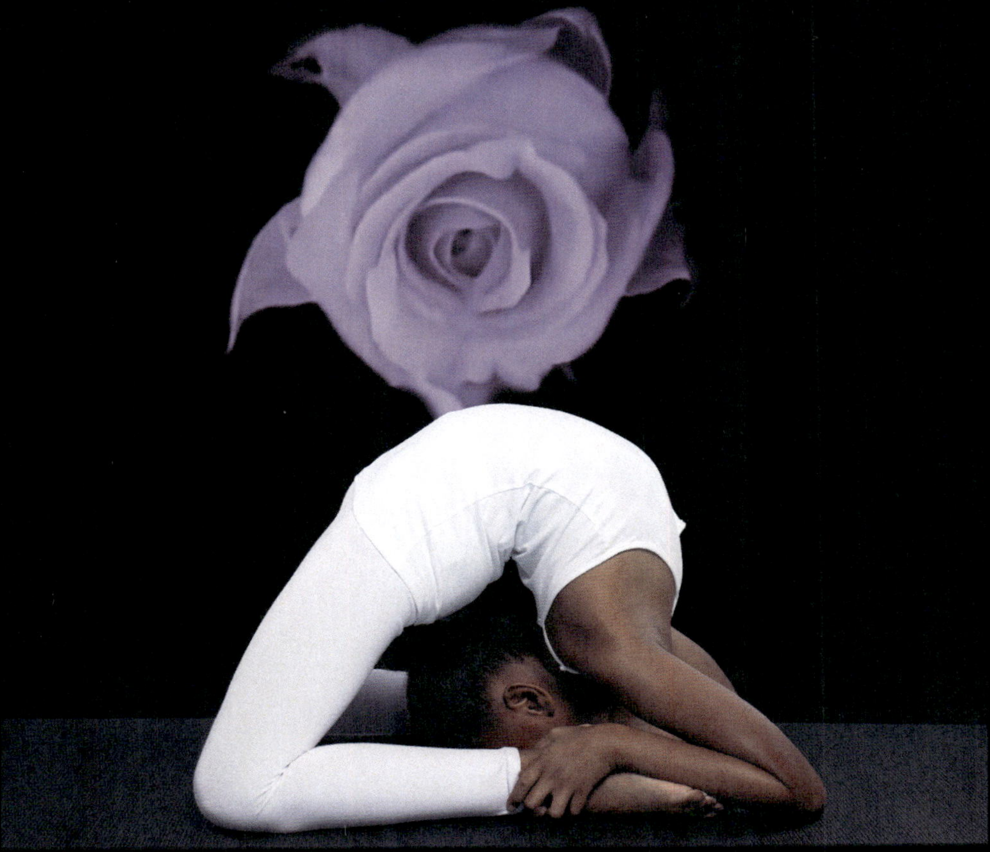

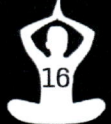

You can look like a Cat in this pose.

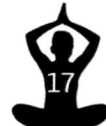

Cat Pose

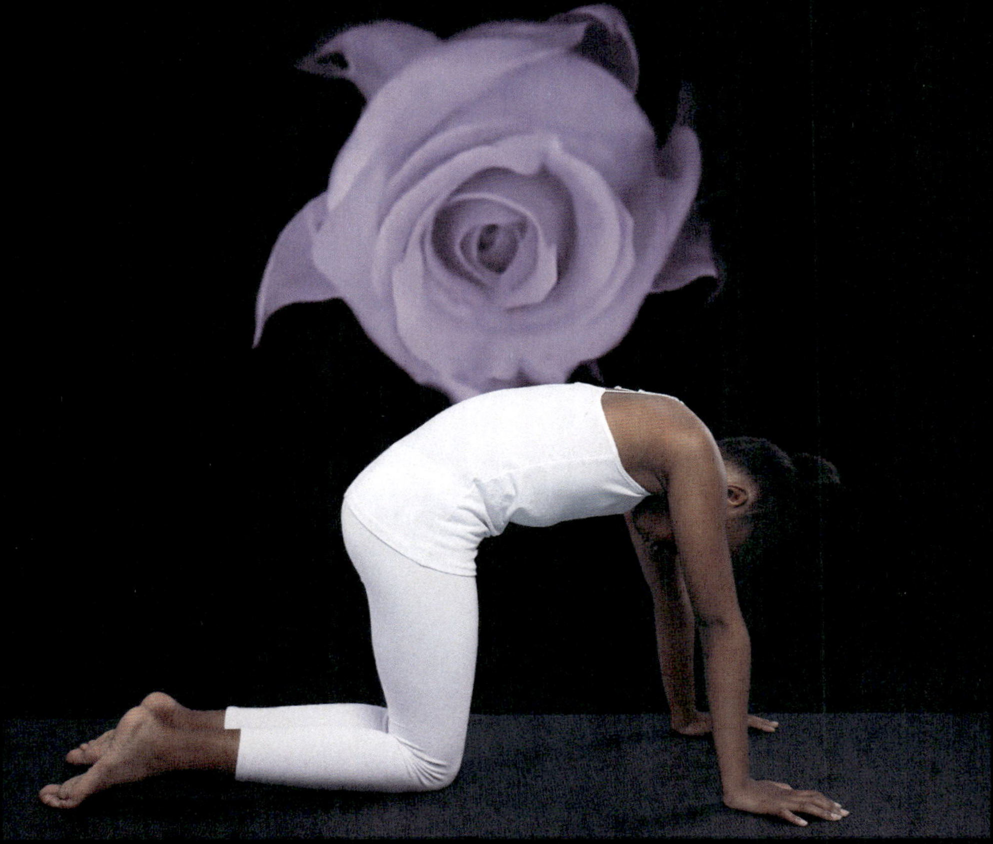

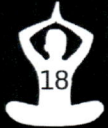

You are doing great!

Try the Downward Facing Dog Pose.

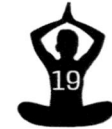

Downward Facing Dog Pose

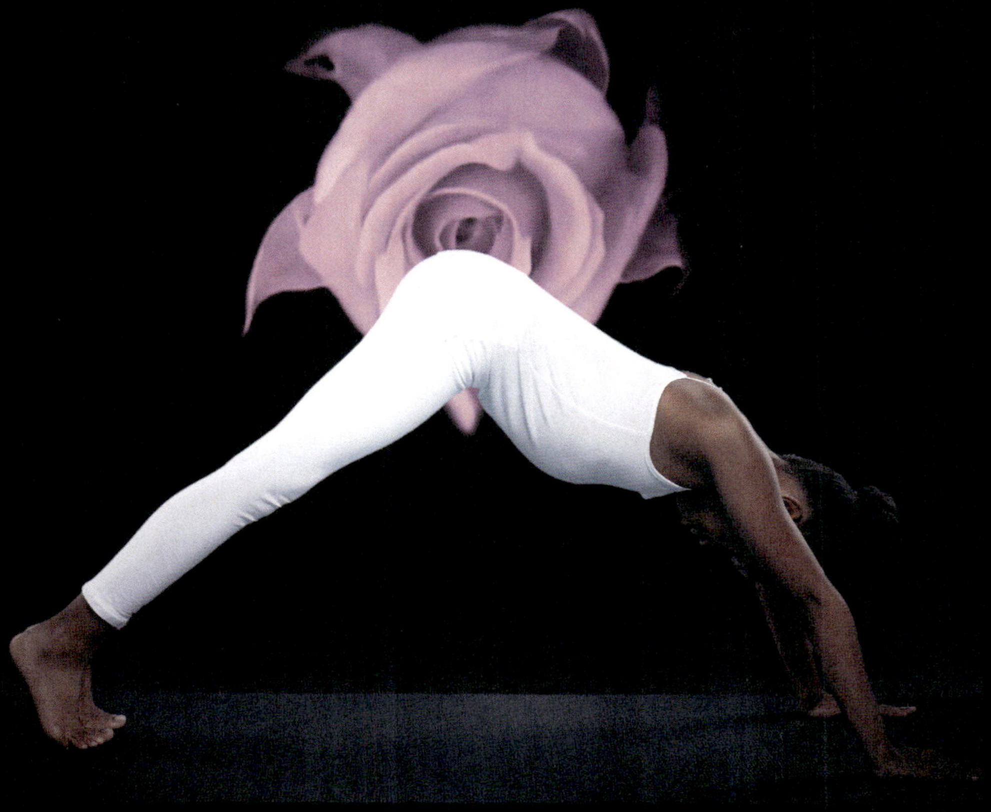

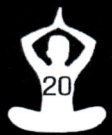

Next, try the Low Lunge Pose.

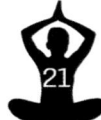

Low Lunge Pose

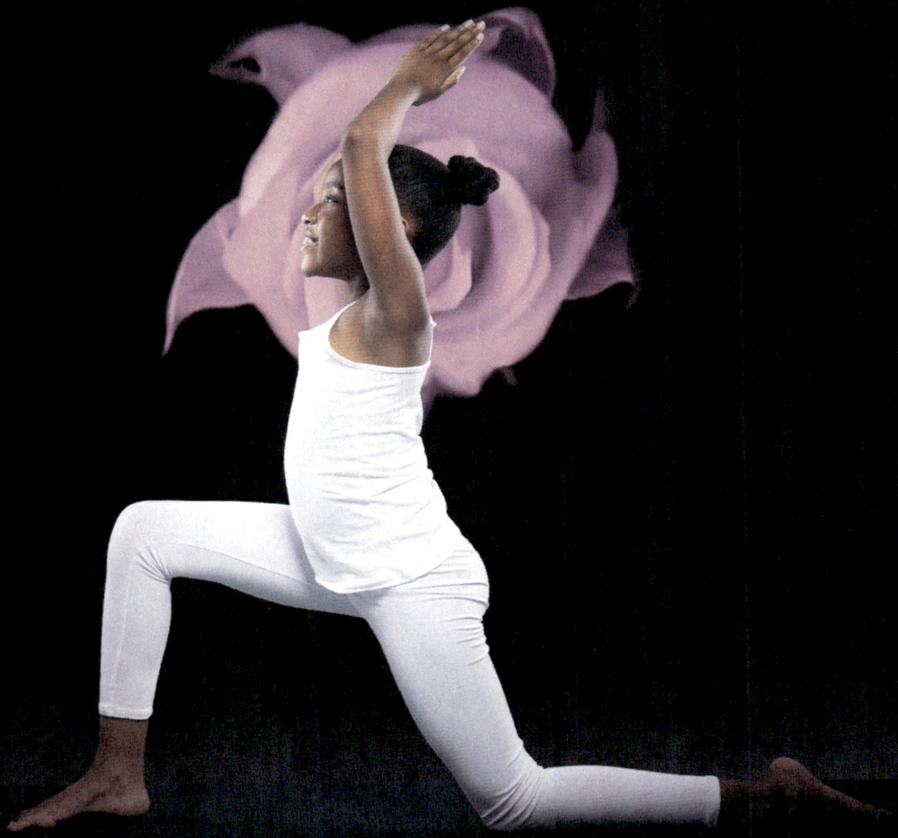

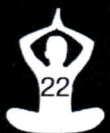

I love the Extended Triangle Pose. Try it with me.

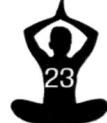

Extended Triangle Pose

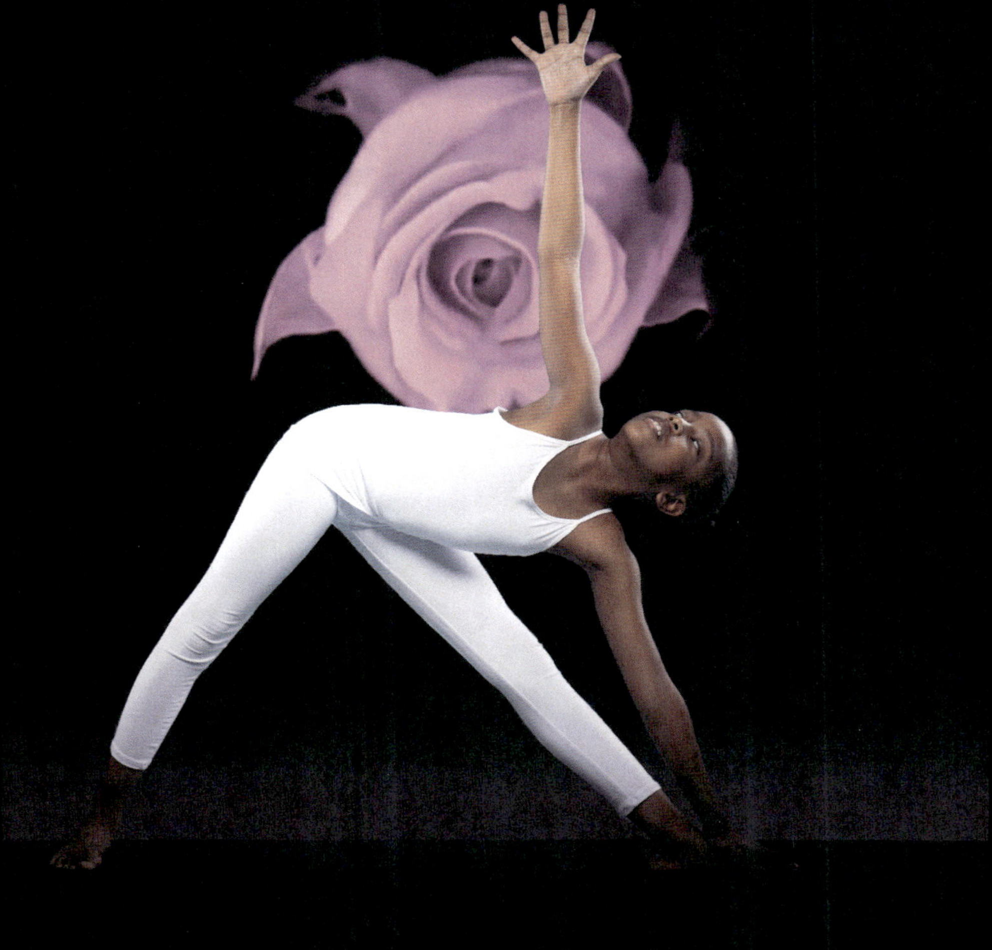

Pose like a warrior. You're so strong!

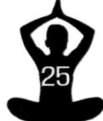

Warrior II Pose

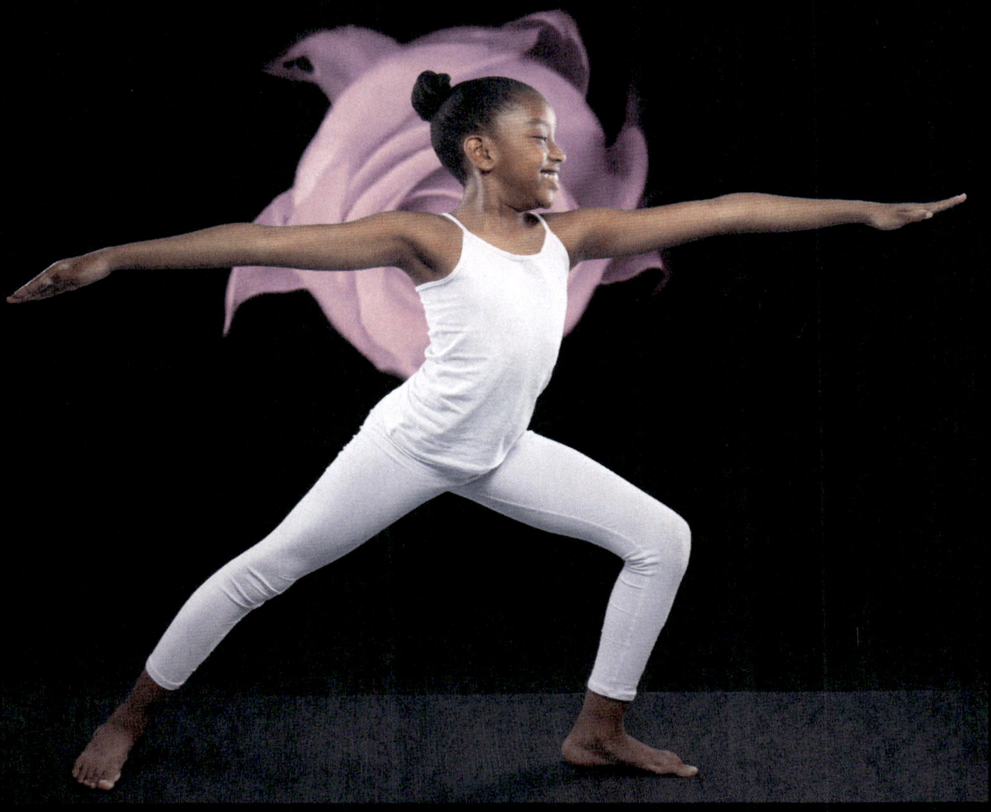

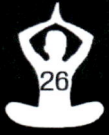

You did amazing!

Now you can show others how to do yoga.

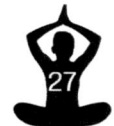

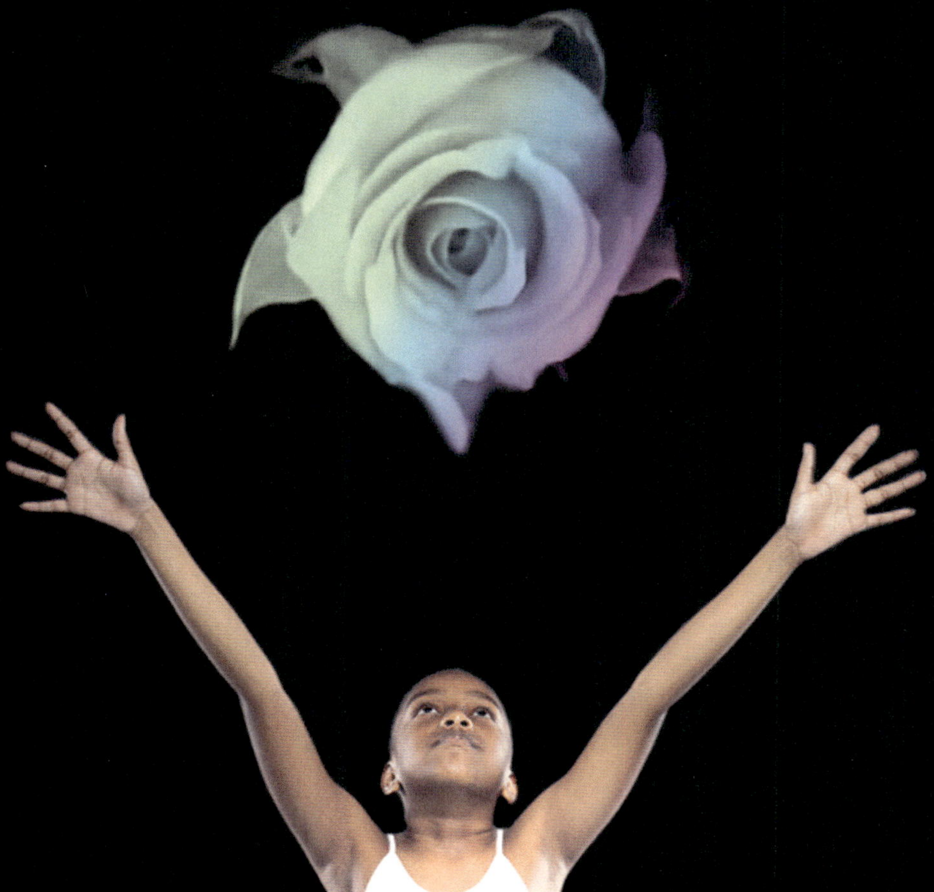

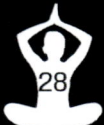

Bio

Abbyelle loves to model, dance and act.

She enjoys recreating pictures and different moves. Join her on her journey.

IG: @abbyelle12
Facebook: The Abby Elle show

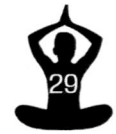

Made in the USA
Middletown, DE
03 June 2024